The Benzodiazepine Withdrawal Journal

Jennifer Austin Leigh, PsyD

This book is not intended as medical advice. This book is intended as information only and is not a tool for diagnosing or treating any illness.
The author is not a licensed M.D. or a licensed psychologist.

Please seek medical attention if you are concerned about your health.
Please seek immediate help if you are suicidal.
The user of this journal is responsible for their decisions/actions and in no way holds the author responsible.

Dedicated to Dr. Heather Ashton.

Actions that nourish the soul —
from Wisdom of Anxiety

- Offering gratitude
- Recording + tending to dreams
- Fresh air + sunshine
- Smiling at a stranger
- Gardening
- Beauty, flowers, color, trees
- Sitting near a body of water or immersing in water
- Walking + talking with a close friend
- Taking the long way home
- Meandering
- Encountering a wild animal
- Pets
- Reading or writing a poem
- Drawing, painting, writing, dancing, singing, c
- Being in nature
- Autumn colors, snowfall, spring buds
- Walking in the rain
- Talking to the moon
- Looking at the stars

- Listening to crickets
- Candlelight
- Baths
- Stillness, silence, & solitude
- Doing less + being more
- Being in silence

Introduction

This journal was created for people who are off of their benzodiazepine and healing. It was created so that you can record your recovery experience. You'll be able to keep track of your symptoms, activities, possible triggers, sleep, diet, exercise, etc., and make notations about your cares or concerns. You can also journal about distractions that work for you as well as explore your spiritual beliefs and practices. You can include anything that is helpful for you to journal about.

You may require more than the number of pages in this book before you feel that you are healed. Please feel free to copy a blank page and make as many copies as you need.

You can share this journal with your doctor, therapist, or anyone you want to better understand what you are experiencing. (There is a section for doctors, therapists, and friends and family should you need to help educate them.)

It may be helpful to work with a doctor or a therapist, but do keep in mind that many are uneducated about benzos and benzo withdrawal and they may offer advice that isn't helpful and could be hurtful. Arm yourself with knowledge so that you can be your own best advocate. Do your research!

Resources

There are many resources available for understanding benzo withdrawal. A simple Google search will reveal many websites dedicated to helping people who are experiencing benzo withdrawal. A search on Facebook will show many groups dedicated to supporting people through benzo withdrawal. These are popular websites

benzobuddies.org

baylissa.com

w-bad.org

benzo.org.uk

benzoinfo.com

benzowithdrawalhelp.com

A word of caution about forums and groups. Although it is helpful to discuss withdrawal symptoms with others who are going through withdrawal, it is not advisable to spend too much time in groups or forums. It can be depressing and make your symptoms feel worse.

Remember, people who have had an easy withdrawal, or who have healed quickly, do not spend their time posting online. They are out enjoying their lives. Only the worst case scenarios are posted online.

Remember too, that your recovery is unique. Don't compare your recovery to the stories you read online.

Distracting

The only way out of benzo withdrawal is through it. Learning to distract from the symptoms is helpful. Engaging your hands and your mind can minimize your focusing on your symptoms. Activities such as painting, gardening, drawing, writing, knitting, sewing, etc., are helpful.

Find an activity that keeps your attention and engage in it as often as you can if you find yourself feeling symptomatic.

Coping Skills

Finding ways to cope with benzo withdrawal symptoms is important. Acceptance, patience, prayer, meditation, a positive attitude, asking for help or support, gentle exercise, yoga, stretching, warm baths, gentle massage, and affirmations are some examples of things that can help in benzo withdrawal.

You can ask others in withdrawal what things have helped them to cope with their symptoms. Please be aware that other medications (even over-the-counter) alcohol, marijuana, vitamins, and supplements may make symptoms worse.

Do and Don't

The basic to do list in benzo withdrawal is to eat clean, (one ingredient, organic foods are best). Get adequate rest, engage in gentle exercise, and maintain a positive outlook. Don't drink alcohol or take supplements, vitamins or any medication that works on GABA (or flares your symptoms). Avoid sugar, processed foods, chemicals, and stress.

Information For Doctors

Benzodiazepines have been on the market for decades. However, it is only with the advent of the internet that information regarding their dangers has become more widely known. Still, many doctors are uneducated about benzodiazepines and harm their patients unwittingly.

Benzodiazepines can cause chemical brain damage in some people, even when taken as prescribed. Benzodiazepines downregulate GABA receptors which in turn cause a myriad of uncomfortable and intense symptoms (and in some extreme cases, life-threatening). Not everyone will be harmed by a benzo, but many are. Withdrawal symptoms can occur even on a steady dose. This is known as tolerance withdrawal. Paradoxical reactions can also occur, causing uncomfortable symptoms.

Benzo withdrawal is a syndrome that includes many symptoms and can mimic MS, Lyme, ALS, OCD, Alzheimer's, Schizoaffective Disorder, Bi-polar Disorder, Borderline Personality Disorder, and Parkinson's. Symptoms can include panic, anxiety, terror, suicide ideation, akathisia, intrusive thoughts, nerve pain, joint pain, muscle pain, hallucinations, dizziness, insomnia, burning, tingling, tinnitus, vomiting, diarrhea, constipation, and more. Symptoms can last months to years after the drug has been discontinued and often wax and wane, commonly known as "windows" and "waves" in the benzo community.

Key Points For The Medical Community

Key points that the medical community must understand in order to help and not harm their patients are

1. Even taken as prescribed, patients can become chemically dependent. Dependency is not addiction. Most people wishing to become benzo free are not addicts in the traditional sense of the word. One does not have to have an "addictive" personality to become dependent on a benzodiazepine. Dependency can occur in a matter of days.

2. Withdrawal symptoms are not the return of any pre-existing condition, nor are they indicative of any new permanent illness.

3. Dose reduction should be no more than ten percent in order to minimize withdrawal symptoms. (It can take months or years to taper safely.)

4. Detox or rehabs are not encouraged as a means to get benzo free as they taper patients off too quickly and they are inclined to add more psych meds, which are usually damaging.

5. Psych meds are usually not helpful in treating benzodiazepine withdrawal. They often make symptoms worse. It is normal to have depression, anxiety, panic, terror, paranoia, intrusive thoughts, guilt/shame, and extreme psychological issues, as well as painful/frightening physical symptoms in withdrawal. Even people who have never presented with any previous psychological issues can experience extreme states in benzo withdrawal. Psychosis is rate, but it does occur. Withdrawal symptoms will gradually disappear on their own. Treating these symptoms is not advised as the medications can increase benzo withdrawal symptoms or create another situation where a drug must be tapered and another withdrawal syndrome experienced.

6. Kindling is a phenomenon that occurs with alcohol, barbiturates, and benzodiazepines. This is why up-dosing is not recommended. It can cause a worsening of withdrawal symptoms.

7. Setbacks can occur once a patient is fully recovered. Setbacks usually happen after taking a medication or drinking alcohol but can also be caused by stressful situations. It can take years for the nervous system to heal completely (even after symptoms are gone) from the damage caused by a benzodiazepine. Medicating setback symptoms can cause a worsening of symptoms.

8. Learning the common dos and don'ts in benzo withdrawal is helpful eat whole (one ingredient) foods, no sugar, caffeine, alcohol, additives, MSG, preservatives or colorings. Vitamin D, B, magnesium, and fish oil can increase symptoms. Herbs or supplements that work on GABA are prohibited (valerian, kava kava, phenibut, chamomile, etc.). Gentle exercise is best as vigorous movements/cardio can increase symptoms. Stressful situations increase withdrawal symptoms and should be avoided.

9. Reinstating after thirty days off of a benzodiazepine is not recommended. It rarely works and most often causes an intensity in symptoms.

10. Never prescribe a fluoroquinolone antibiotic to anyone taking a benzodiazepine. It can cause a cold-turkey reaction.

11. The only known cure for benzo withdrawal is time. Medications do not cure withdrawal and many make symptoms worse.

Information For Therapists

Therapists who are uneducated about the withdrawal syndrome can unwittingly harm their patients. It is important to understand withdrawal in order to best serve your patients.

A patient in benzodiazepine withdrawal may present with a myriad of disorders. These are not organic illnesses and will abate on their own in time. It is best to not treat these symptoms or to recommend medication at the hands of a psychiatrist as medications very often make matters worse and they usually do not reduce the intensity of symptoms.

Anxiety, fear, panic, terror, agitation, depression, extreme paranoia, insomnia, intrusive thoughts, looping thoughts, OCD thinking/behaviors, hallucinations, delusions, bi-polar thinking/behavior, suicide ideation, akathisia, tinnitus, as well as a myriad of painful and frightening physical symptoms are very common in benzo withdrawal. Reassuring your patient that their symptoms will go away on their own is helpful. Diagnosing someone in benzo withdrawal as having a psychological disorder is not helpful and often hurtful to the patient.

People experiencing benzo withdrawal do not have the ability to relive and reintegrate old trauma, and to insist that they talk about such things puts them at risk for becoming more symptomatic. They may be plagued with regrets, sorrow, or shame from the past (known in the benzo community as life-review) but this is a common withdrawal symptom and will go away in time.

There are no therapies that will help GABA receptors heal faster. Time is the only known cure for benzo withdrawal. Compassionate support to help a patient cope with withdrawal symptoms is the best approach.

Information For Friends And Family

This is reprinted from benzowithdrawalhelp.com

If we had been diagnosed with cancer, our family and friends would know that we are sick. They'd make us casseroles, take us to our chemo appointments, and call us to see how we are doing. After all, cancer is a serious matter, *They would be concerned.* But family and friends have very little knowledge about benzo withdrawal so they don't know *just how serious it is.* This is what we wish they knew about benzo withdrawal.

We trusted our doctors and took a pill, as prescribed, and it damaged one of the two main "circuit boards" that regulate our brains. We have damaged GABA receptors, which means our bodies and minds don't have the ability to slow/calm down. We suffer from chemical brain damage that can take a long time (sometimes years) to heal. Many of us have severe physical symptoms painful joints, bones, muscles, teeth, eyes, mouth, etc. Our skin burns. It feels as if we have bugs crawling under our skin, or that bees are stinging us. Our muscles twitch and spasm. Our legs are weak and our balance is off; walking is difficult. But some of us do walk, and walk, and walk, as we are suffering from akathisia, a movement disorder that causes an inner restlessness and a compelling need to be in constant motion. We have painful and frightening pressure in our heads, making it feel as if the world is sloshing around us. Many of us are bedridden for months at a time, unable to take care of the most basic of human needs. We can't think properly, and our memory is impaired. There are countless other physical symptoms that we may have as this is not an exhaustive list. What we want our friends and family to know is that we are sick and in pain. It's hard to manage our lives. Many of us are unable to work or to function in our roles and duties as a parent. On top of being physically sick, we have mental symptoms as well.

Without a functioning GABA system to calm the fight/flight/freeze response of our brains, we live in a state of fear, anxiety, paranoia, or terror. We may have depersonalization or derealization. Frequent panic attacks are common. In benzo withdrawal, we lose the ability to feel positive emotions. Love, happiness, and joy are not within our reach. We slog through our days feeling a zombie-like doom and gloom. Intrusive and looping thoughts are common. We have very little control over our minds. Visual, auditory, and olfactory hallucinations are not uncommon. We wish that our friends and family understood how frightening it is to lose the ability to think rationally and to no longer feel as if you are the same person you were before benzo withdrawal. It is hard to live in the altered reality that benzo withdrawal can create.

We want friends and family to know that we are scared and oftentimes feeling hopeless. We need a great deal of reassurance. When we get scared that we will never get well; that we will never be ourselves again, we want you to remind us that we are healing. We know that we tax your patience, and we feel bad about being so needy. But we hope that you can hang in there with us as we do the hard work of holding on and surviving. We want you to take care of yourself so that you have the energy to take care of us too when we need your help. Please don't burn out! It's okay to take time away from us to refresh and recharge.

We know that the only cure for benzo withdrawal is time, so your suggestions to "Go see a doctor" or "Get back on your meds," or "Up your dose," doesn't help us. See, what you don't know is that the medical community understands very little about the damage these drugs cause. We've learned from thousands of others who have lived through benzo withdrawal. There are no meds for withdrawal, nor should anyone be on a benzo for more than a few days. Please trust that we have educated ourselves about the healing process from benzos.

We want our friends and family to know that benzo withdrawal will come to an end one day, (even if we don't believe that ourselves). Our brains and our bodies will heal. We will start new chapters in our lives. We want everyone that we love to go the distance with us and to celebrate the dawning of the new day when we are recovered. Until then, we just need you to listen to us, to be there for us. We don't need you to try to fix us; we know that you can't. Just love us, exactly as we are, and where we are on our journey. We thank you and love you for being there for us while we battle an invisible, and medically ignored illness of great magnitude.

There is hardly anything of our lives that is recognizable in benzo withdrawal. We are doing the best we can with what we have to work with. We can't magically think "happy thoughts," or "snap out of it." We have to wait for our brains to heal. Please, wait with us.

Basic Information:

Current Medications

Please list your current medications and doses

Emergency Contacts/Doctors

Please list names, telephone numbers, addresses

My Support Team

Please list people you trust to help you through benzo withdrawal

My Positive Decision(s)

I am making the decision(s) to

Withdrawal Journal

In the next section you can record the date, your symptoms, your sleep pattern, distractions, diet, exercise, emotional support systems, spiritual beliefs (prayers, meditations) questions or concerns, etc. (If you are taking any other medication, you can note them in your journal.) You are encouraged to write a positive affirmation that is written in the present tense, is powerful and positive. Example. "I am healing."

The journal has one page of prompts and a blank page for your thoughts, scribbles, notes, sketches, etc. Be as creative as you want to be!

Date:

Sleep:

Diet/Nutrition:

Exercise:

Distractions:

Spiritual Practice:

Withdrawal Symptoms:

Concerns:

Positive Affirmation:

Goals, Dreams, Wisdom, Inspiration:

Date:

Sleep:

Diet/Nutrition:

Exercise:

Distractions:

Spiritual Practice:

Withdrawal Symptoms:

Concerns:

Positive Affirmation:

Goals, Dreams, Wisdom, Inspiration:

Date:

Sleep:

Diet/Nutrition:

Exercise:

Distractions:

Spiritual Practice:

Withdrawal Symptoms:

Concerns:

Positive Affirmation:

Goals, Dreams, Wisdom, Inspiration:

Date:

Sleep:

Diet/Nutrition:

Exercise:

Distractions:

Spiritual Practice:

Withdrawal Symptoms:

Concerns:

Positive Affirmation:

Goals, Dreams, Wisdom, Inspiration:

Date:

Sleep:

Diet/Nutrition:

Exercise:

Distractions:

Spiritual Practice:

Withdrawal Symptoms:

Concerns:

Positive Affirmation:

Goals, Dreams, Wisdom, Inspiration:

Date:

Sleep:

Diet/Nutrition:

Exercise:

Distractions:

Spiritual Practice:

Withdrawal Symptoms:

Concerns:

Positive Affirmation:

Goals, Dreams, Wisdom, Inspiration:

Date:

Sleep:

Diet/Nutrition:

Exercise:

Distractions:

Spiritual Practice:

Withdrawal Symptoms:

Concerns:

Positive Affirmation:

Goals, Dreams, Wisdom, Inspiration:

Date:

Sleep:

Diet/Nutrition:

Exercise:

Distractions:

Spiritual Practice:

Withdrawal Symptoms:

Concerns:

Positive Affirmation:

Goals, Dreams, Wisdom, Inspiration:

Date:

Sleep:

Diet/Nutrition:

Exercise:

Distractions:

Spiritual Practice:

Withdrawal Symptoms:

Concerns:

Positive Affirmation:

Goals, Dreams, Wisdom, Inspiration:

Date:

Sleep:

Diet/Nutrition:

Exercise:

Distractions:

Spiritual Practice:

Withdrawal Symptoms:

Concerns:

Positive Affirmation:

Goals, Dreams, Wisdom, Inspiration:

Date:

Sleep:

Diet/Nutrition:

Exercise:

Distractions:

Spiritual Practice:

Withdrawal Symptoms:

Concerns:

Positive Affirmation:

Goals, Dreams, Wisdom, Inspiration:

Date:

Sleep:

Diet/Nutrition:

Exercise:

Distractions:

Spiritual Practice:

Withdrawal Symptoms:

Concerns:

Positive Affirmation:

Goals, Dreams, Wisdom, Inspiration:

Date:

Sleep:

Diet/Nutrition:

Exercise:

Distractions:

Spiritual Practice:

Withdrawal Symptoms:

Concerns:

Positive Affirmation:

Goals, Dreams, Wisdom, Inspiration:

Date:

Sleep:

Diet/Nutrition:

Exercise:

Distractions:

Spiritual Practice:

Withdrawal Symptoms:

Concerns:

Positive Affirmation:

Goals, Dreams, Wisdom, Inspiration:

Date:

Sleep:

Diet/Nutrition:

Exercise:

Distractions:

Spiritual Practice:

Withdrawal Symptoms:

Concerns:

Positive Affirmation:

Goals, Dreams, Wisdom, Inspiration:

Date:

Sleep:

Diet/Nutrition:

Exercise:

Distractions:

Spiritual Practice:

Withdrawal Symptoms:

Concerns:

Positive Affirmation:

Goals, Dreams, Wisdom, Inspiration:

Date:

Sleep:

Diet/Nutrition:

Exercise:

Distractions:

Spiritual Practice:

Withdrawal Symptoms:

Concerns:

Positive Affirmation:

Goals, Dreams, Wisdom, Inspiration:

Date:

Sleep:

Diet/Nutrition:

Exercise:

Distractions:

Spiritual Practice:

Withdrawal Symptoms:

Concerns:

Positive Affirmation:

Goals, Dreams, Wisdom, Inspiration:

Date:

Sleep:

Diet/Nutrition:

Exercise:

Distractions:

Spiritual Practice:

Withdrawal Symptoms:

Concerns:

Positive Affirmation:

Goals, Dreams, Wisdom, Inspiration:

Date:

Sleep:

Diet/Nutrition:

Exercise:

Distractions:

Spiritual Practice:

Withdrawal Symptoms:

Concerns:

Positive Affirmation:

Goals, Dreams, Wisdom, Inspiration:

Date:

Sleep:

Diet/Nutrition:

Exercise:

Distractions:

Spiritual Practice:

Withdrawal Symptoms:

Concerns:

Positive Affirmation:

Goals, Dreams, Wisdom, Inspiration:

Date:

Sleep:

Diet/Nutrition:

Exercise:

Distractions:

Spiritual Practice:

Withdrawal Symptoms:

Concerns:

Positive Affirmation:

Goals, Dreams, Wisdom, Inspiration:

Date:

Sleep:

Diet/Nutrition:

Exercise:

Distractions:

Spiritual Practice:

Withdrawal Symptoms:

Concerns:

Positive Affirmation:

Goals, Dreams, Wisdom, Inspiration:

Date:

Sleep:

Diet/Nutrition:

Exercise:

Distractions:

Spiritual Practice:

Withdrawal Symptoms:

Concerns:

Positive Affirmation:

Goals, Dreams, Wisdom, Inspiration:

Date:

Sleep:

Diet/Nutrition:

Exercise:

Distractions:

Spiritual Practice:

Withdrawal Symptoms:

Concerns:

Positive Affirmation:

Goals, Dreams, Wisdom, Inspiration:

Date:

Sleep:

Diet/Nutrition:

Exercise:

Distractions:

Spiritual Practice:

Withdrawal Symptoms:

Concerns:

Positive Affirmation:

Goals, Dreams, Wisdom, Inspiration:

Date:

Sleep:

Diet/Nutrition:

Exercise:

Distractions:

Spiritual Practice:

Withdrawal Symptoms:

Concerns:

Positive Affirmation:

Goals, Dreams, Wisdom, Inspiration:

Date:

Sleep:

Diet/Nutrition:

Exercise:

Distractions:

Spiritual Practice:

Withdrawal Symptoms:

Concerns:

Positive Affirmation:

Goals, Dreams, Wisdom, Inspiration:

Date:

Sleep:

Diet/Nutrition:

Exercise:

Distractions:

Spiritual Practice:

Withdrawal Symptoms:

Concerns:

Positive Affirmation:

Goals, Dreams, Wisdom, Inspiration:

Date:

Sleep:

Diet/Nutrition:

Exercise:

Distractions:

Spiritual Practice:

Withdrawal Symptoms:

Concerns:

Positive Affirmation:

Goals, Dreams, Wisdom, Inspiration:

Date:

Sleep:

Diet/Nutrition:

Exercise:

Distractions:

Spiritual Practice:

Withdrawal Symptoms:

Concerns:

Positive Affirmation:

Goals, Dreams, Wisdom, Inspiration:

Date:

Sleep:

Diet/Nutrition:

Exercise:

Distractions:

Spiritual Practice:

Withdrawal Symptoms:

Concerns:

Positive Affirmation:

Goals, Dreams, Wisdom, Inspiration:

Date:

Sleep:

Diet/Nutrition:

Exercise:

Distractions:

Spiritual Practice:

Withdrawal Symptoms:

Concerns:

Positive Affirmation:

Goals, Dreams, Wisdom, Inspiration:

Date:

Sleep:

Diet/Nutrition:

Exercise:

Distractions:

Spiritual Practice:

Withdrawal Symptoms:

Concerns:

Positive Affirmation:

Goals, Dreams, Wisdom, Inspiration:

Date:

Sleep:

Diet/Nutrition:

Exercise:

Distractions:

Spiritual Practice:

Withdrawal Symptoms:

Concerns:

Positive Affirmation:

Goals, Dreams, Wisdom, Inspiration:

Date:

Sleep:

Diet/Nutrition:

Exercise:

Distractions:

Spiritual Practice:

Withdrawal Symptoms:

Concerns:

Positive Affirmation:

Goals, Dreams, Wisdom, Inspiration:

Date:

Sleep:

Diet/Nutrition:

Exercise:

Distractions:

Spiritual Practice:

Withdrawal Symptoms:

Concerns:

Positive Affirmation:

Goals, Dreams, Wisdom, Inspiration:

Date:

Sleep:

Diet/Nutrition:

Exercise:

Distractions:

Spiritual Practice:

Withdrawal Symptoms:

Concerns:

Positive Affirmation:

Goals, Dreams, Wisdom, Inspiration:

Date:

Sleep:

Diet/Nutrition:

Exercise:

Distractions:

Spiritual Practice:

Withdrawal Symptoms:

Concerns:

Positive Affirmation:

Goals, Dreams, Wisdom, Inspiration:

Date:

Sleep:

Diet/Nutrition:

Exercise:

Distractions:

Spiritual Practice:

Withdrawal Symptoms:

Concerns:

Positive Affirmation:

Goals, Dreams, Wisdom, Inspiration:

Date:

Sleep:

Diet/Nutrition:

Exercise:

Distractions:

Spiritual Practice:

Withdrawal Symptoms:

Concerns:

Positive Affirmation:

Goals, Dreams, Wisdom, Inspiration:

Date:

Sleep:

Diet/Nutrition:

Exercise:

Distractions:

Spiritual Practice:

Withdrawal Symptoms:

Concerns:

Positive Affirmation:

Goals, Dreams, Wisdom, Inspiration:

Date:

Sleep:

Diet/Nutrition:

Exercise:

Distractions:

Spiritual Practice:

Withdrawal Symptoms:

Concerns:

Positive Affirmation:

Goals, Dreams, Wisdom, Inspiration:

Date:

Sleep:

Diet/Nutrition:

Exercise:

Distractions:

Spiritual Practice:

Withdrawal Symptoms:

Concerns:

Positive Affirmation:

Goals, Dreams, Wisdom, Inspiration:

Date:

Sleep:

Diet/Nutrition:

Exercise:

Distractions:

Spiritual Practice:

Withdrawal Symptoms:

Concerns:

Positive Affirmation:

Goals, Dreams, Wisdom, Inspiration:

Date:

Sleep:

Diet/Nutrition:

Exercise:

Distractions:

Spiritual Practice:

Withdrawal Symptoms:

Concerns:

Positive Affirmation:

Goals, Dreams, Wisdom, Inspiration:

Date:

Sleep:

Diet/Nutrition:

Exercise:

Distractions:

Spiritual Practice:

Withdrawal Symptoms:

Concerns:

Positive Affirmation:

Goals, Dreams, Wisdom, Inspiration:

Date:

Sleep:

Diet/Nutrition:

Exercise:

Distractions:

Spiritual Practice:

Withdrawal Symptoms:

Concerns:

Positive Affirmation:

Goals, Dreams, Wisdom, Inspiration:

Date:

Sleep:

Diet/Nutrition:

Exercise:

Distractions:

Spiritual Practice:

Withdrawal Symptoms:

Concerns:

Positive Affirmation:

Goals, Dreams, Wisdom, Inspiration:

Date:

Sleep:

Diet/Nutrition:

Exercise:

Distractions:

Spiritual Practice:

Withdrawal Symptoms:

Concerns:

Positive Affirmation:

Goals, Dreams, Wisdom, Inspiration:

Date:

Sleep:

Diet/Nutrition:

Exercise:

Distractions:

Spiritual Practice:

Withdrawal Symptoms:

Concerns:

Positive Affirmation:

Goals, Dreams, Wisdom, Inspiration:

Date:

Sleep:

Diet/Nutrition:

Exercise:

Distractions:

Spiritual Practice:

Withdrawal Symptoms:

Concerns:

Positive Affirmation:

Goals, Dreams, Wisdom, Inspiration:

Date:

Sleep:

Diet/Nutrition:

Exercise:

Distractions:

Spiritual Practice:

Withdrawal Symptoms:

Concerns:

Positive Affirmation:

Goals, Dreams, Wisdom, Inspiration:

Date:

Sleep:

Diet/Nutrition:

Exercise:

Distractions:

Spiritual Practice:

Withdrawal Symptoms:

Concerns:

Positive Affirmation:

Goals, Dreams, Wisdom, Inspiration:

Date:

Sleep:

Diet/Nutrition:

Exercise:

Distractions:

Spiritual Practice:

Withdrawal Symptoms:

Concerns:

Positive Affirmation:

Goals, Dreams, Wisdom, Inspiration:

Date:

Sleep:

Diet/Nutrition:

Exercise:

Distractions:

Spiritual Practice:

Withdrawal Symptoms:

Concerns:

Positive Affirmation:

Goals, Dreams, Wisdom, Inspiration:

Date:

Sleep:

Diet/Nutrition:

Exercise:

Distractions:

Spiritual Practice:

Withdrawal Symptoms:

Concerns:

Positive Affirmation:

Goals, Dreams, Wisdom, Inspiration:

Date:

Sleep:

Diet/Nutrition:

Exercise:

Distractions:

Spiritual Practice:

Withdrawal Symptoms:

Concerns:

Positive Affirmation:

Goals, Dreams, Wisdom, Inspiration:

Date:

Sleep:

Diet/Nutrition:

Exercise:

Distractions:

Spiritual Practice:

Withdrawal Symptoms:

Concerns:

Positive Affirmation:

Goals, Dreams, Wisdom, Inspiration:

Date:

Sleep:

Diet/Nutrition:

Exercise:

Distractions:

Spiritual Practice:

Withdrawal Symptoms:

Concerns:

Positive Affirmation:

Goals, Dreams, Wisdom, Inspiration:

Date:

Sleep:

Diet/Nutrition:

Exercise:

Distractions:

Spiritual Practice:

Withdrawal Symptoms:

Concerns:

Positive Affirmation:

Goals, Dreams, Wisdom, Inspiration:

Date:

Sleep:

Diet/Nutrition:

Exercise:

Distractions:

Spiritual Practice:

Withdrawal Symptoms:

Concerns:

Positive Affirmation:

Goals, Dreams, Wisdom, Inspiration:

Date:

Sleep:

Diet/Nutrition:

Exercise:

Distractions:

Spiritual Practice:

Withdrawal Symptoms:

Concerns:

Positive Affirmation:

Goals, Dreams, Wisdom, Inspiration:

Date:

Sleep:

Diet/Nutrition:

Exercise:

Distractions:

Spiritual Practice:

Withdrawal Symptoms:

Concerns:

Positive Affirmation:

Goals, Dreams, Wisdom, Inspiration:

Date:

Sleep:

Diet/Nutrition:

Exercise:

Distractions:

Spiritual Practice:

Withdrawal Symptoms:

Concerns:

Positive Affirmation:

Goals, Dreams, Wisdom, Inspiration:

Date:

Sleep:

Diet/Nutrition:

Exercise:

Distractions:

Spiritual Practice:

Withdrawal Symptoms:

Concerns:

Positive Affirmation:

Goals, Dreams, Wisdom, Inspiration:

Date:

Sleep:

Diet/Nutrition:

Exercise:

Distractions:

Spiritual Practice:

Withdrawal Symptoms:

Concerns:

Positive Affirmation:

Goals, Dreams, Wisdom, Inspiration: